Prostate Health

A Guide to Cancer Survival

Roy Kadan

Introduction:

Welcome to "Empowering Prostate Health: A Guide to Cancer Survival," a comprehensive and accessible resource designed to empower individuals with knowledge and strategies to navigate the complex landscape of prostate health and cancer survival. In the pages that follow, we embark on a journey to understand the intricacies of the prostate, explore common health issues, and delve into proactive measures for prevention and early detection.

Chapter by chapter, we will address key aspects of prostate health, providing in-depth insights and practical guidance. From understanding the anatomy and function of the prostate to exploring the intricacies of a prostate cancer diagnosis, this book aims to demystify complex medical concepts and make them accessible to readers of all backgrounds.

Through the course of this guide, we will not only discuss the medical aspects of prostate health but also delve into the lifestyle choices and proactive measures that contribute to overall well-being. From the importance of regular check-ups to the role of nutrition, exercise, and mental health, we will equip you with the tools needed to make informed decisions about your prostate health.

Navigating a prostate cancer diagnosis can be overwhelming, and our book is designed to be a supportive companion on this journey. We will explore various treatment options, manage side effects, and discuss strategies for maintaining a positive mindset throughout the process.

Additionally, we'll shed light on life beyond prostate cancer, emphasizing the importance of post-treatment care and survivorship.

"Empowering Prostate Health" goes beyond providing information; it encourages advocacy, awareness, and community support. As we delve into the latest research and innovations, we aim to inspire individuals to become advocates for their own health and contribute to the collective effort in the fight against prostate cancer.

Throughout this guide, you will find real-life stories of prostate cancer survivors, offering inspiration and hope. Their journeys illustrate the resilience of the human spirit and serve as a testament to the progress made in prostate cancer treatment and survivorship.

By the end of this book, you will not only possess a comprehensive understanding of prostate health and cancer survival but also feel empowered to take charge of your well-being. Whether you are navigating a prostate cancer diagnosis or proactively seeking ways to maintain optimal prostate health, this guide is here to support you every step of the way. Let's embark on this journey together, embracing knowledge, empowerment, and resilience in the face of prostate health challenges.

Disclaimer: I am not a medical professional, and this information should not be taken as medical advice. Please consult with a qualified healthcare provider for any questions or concerns regarding your prostate health......By the end of this book, one can possess a thorough understanding of prostate health and cancer survival but also feel empowered to take charge of your well-being.

Contents

Chapter 1

Understanding the Prostate

Anatomy and Function

Tips for Keeping Your Prostate Healthy

The prostate is a small gland located below a man's bladder. It produces fluid that nourishes and transports sperm. As men age, prostate issues like enlargement or cancer become more common. Making certain healthy lifestyle choices can help maintain better prostate function over the years.

Know Your Prostate

Gaining familiarity with this walnut-sized gland enables you to understand warning signs if problems arise. The prostate surrounds the first inch or so of the urethra which carries urine and semen through the penis. Nerves next to the prostate facilitate erections too.

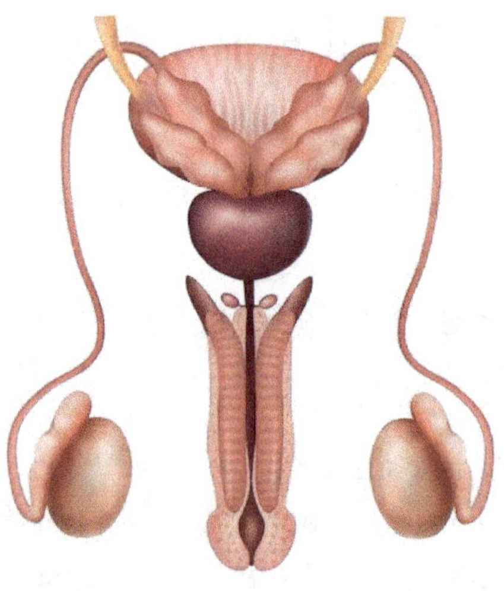

When functioning well, it operates unnoticed delivering nutrients to sperm. When inflamed or overgrown, bothersome urinary or sexual symptoms start interfering with normal activity.

Stay Proactive with Screenings

Without symptoms initially, problems fester

unseen. That's why cancer screening is vital. Guidelines suggest:

- Ages 45-49: Discuss screenings with your doctor
- Ages 50+: Have annual PSA blood tests and physical prostate exams

Testing establishes base lines and detects developing issues for the earliest, most treatable action. Screenings leading to early cancer diagnosis make cure odds over 95-100% based on low-risk tumors.

Maintain a Healthy Diet

Nutritious whole foods provide antioxidants and compounds that reduce inflammation and protect prostate health. Great choices include:

- Tomatoes and tomato sauce
- Cruciferous vegetables
- Soy foods like tofu or edamame
- Oily fish high in omega-3s
- Nuts and seeds
- Green tea
- Berries

- Avocados

These selections may help prevent enlarged prostate and prostate cancer too. Stay hydrated with water and reduce sugary drinks and excessive alcohol.

Keep Physically Active

Move more through aerobic, weight-bearing, and muscle-strengthening exercises most days. Physically active men have lower PSA levels. Combining cardio, core training, and resistance workouts protects prostate health as you age. Aim for 30 minutes daily.

Achieve or Maintain a Healthy Weight

Carrying excess body fat drives inflammation, insulin resistance, and hormone changes that impact cancer and prostate risks. Reach or preserve a moderate weight through calorie-conscious eating and frequent exercise. Just losing 5-10% of weight offers benefits.

Prioritize Stress Management

Chronic stress elevates cortisol and lowers

protective testosterone. This hormonal imbalance makes prostate disorders more likely. Bolster resilience through sufficient sleep, relaxation practices like meditation or yoga, talking therapy, breathing exercises, etc. Listen to your mind and body.

Consider Targeted Supplements

Research indicates certain vitamins, minerals, and plant concentrates may help prostate health. Speak to your doctor about possible advantages of supplements, including:

- Vitamin D and E
- Selenium
- Green tea extracts
- Soy isoflavone pills
- Omega-3 fish oil capsules
- Pumpkin seed extracts
- Zinc and magnesium

Stay alert for urinary or sexual dysfunction red flags requiring prompt evaluation too. Prioritizing healthy lifestyle measures promotes optimal lifelong prostate function.

Chapter 2

Prostate infection signs

Understanding Prostate Infection Signs

The prostate is a small gland located below the bladder in men. It produces fluid that nourishes and protects sperm. An enlarged or inflamed prostate can cause uncomfortable urinary and sexual symptoms. A prostate infection, also called prostatitis, causes these prostate problems.

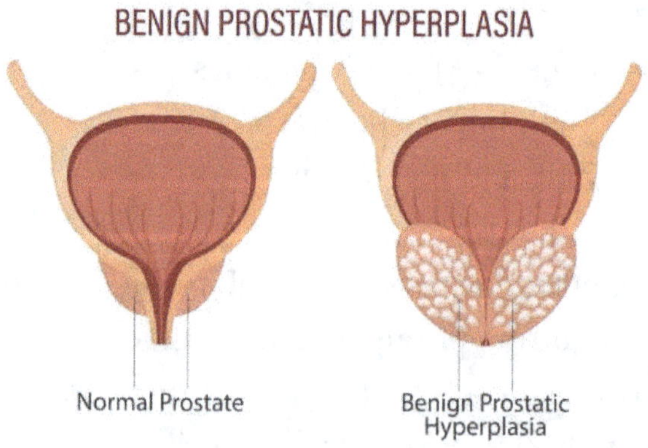

What Causes a Prostate Infection?

Germs like bacteria, viruses, or fungi often cause infectious prostatitis. These germs may get into the prostate from the urethra or through the bloodstream. Sometimes the cause is unknown.

Risk factors for developing an infected prostate include:

- Having a urinary tract infection
- Having an STD
- Recent prostate biopsy or medical procedure
- Weakened immune system
- Structural prostate issues
- Use of urinary catheter

Common Signs of a Prostate Infection

The signs of a prostate infection often involve changes in urinary habits and sexual function. Symptoms may develop slowly or come on suddenly. They include:

- Difficult and Painful Urination

- Burning feeling when urinating
- Frequent need to urinate, sometimes urgently
- Blood in urine or semen
- Dribbling urine or trouble starting a stream
- Straining to empty the bladder
- Feeling the bladder isn't fully emptied
- Pain and Discomfort
- Pain or tenderness in the lower back, abdomen, groin, or rectal area
- Pelvic pain that comes and goes
- Body chills and fever suggest infection
- Sexual Difficulties
- Pain during or after ejaculation
- Blood in semen
- Erectile dysfunction
- Reduced sex drive

Mild cases may have very subtle symptoms or none. Seek medical advice for any persistent urinary or pelvic changes.

Types of Prostatitis

There are four classifications of prostatitis according to causes and symptoms:

- **Acute Bacterial Prostatitis**
  Caused by a bacterial infection, this type of prostatitis comes on suddenly. Symptoms are severe and include chills, fever, nausea, and vomiting. Antibiotics are used to treat it.

- **Chronic Bacterial Prostatitis**
  Ongoing urinary difficulties caused by recurrent prostate infections signify this condition. It is diagnosed through lab tests. Antibiotics and lifestyle changes help manage it.

- **Chronic Nonbacterial Prostatitis**
  This involves long-term pelvic pain and urinary problems without evidence of a bacterial infection. Causes involve nerves or muscles. Treatments aim to ease pain and inflammation.

- **Asymptomatic Inflammatory Prostatitis**
  No symptoms are present with this type, but signs of prostate inflammation or

infection appear on lab tests. Treatment may not be needed but follow-up checks are done.

Seeing a Doctor

Schedule an appointment with a primary care doctor or urologist if you have any symptoms of a possible prostate problem. They will examine you and may order lab tests on urine or prostatic fluid samples. Imaging tests can also check for issues.

Catching and treating prostate infections early helps prevent problems like abscesses or prostate stones from developing later. Though symptoms may come and go, it's best to get persistent prostate issues fully evaluated. Controlling any infection also helps reduce the transmission of bacteria to partners.

Chapter 3

Enlarged Prostate Treatments

Treating an Enlarged Prostate (Benign Prostatic Hyperplasia)

Dealing with an Enlarged Prostate as You Age As men get older, our prostates often get bigger. This happens to lots of guys, even healthy men. Doctors call the condition "benign prostatic hyperplasia", or BPH for short. Basically, it means your prostate gland gets enlarged but isn't cancerous.

What Goes Wrong

Your prostate is about the size of a walnut and sits under your bladder, wrapped around the tube that carries pee out of your body (the urethra). When your prostate gets bigger, it can squeeze that tube making it harder for you to pee normally. The reasons why some men get

BPH and others don't aren't fully clear. It seems to run in families though and happens more as we age.

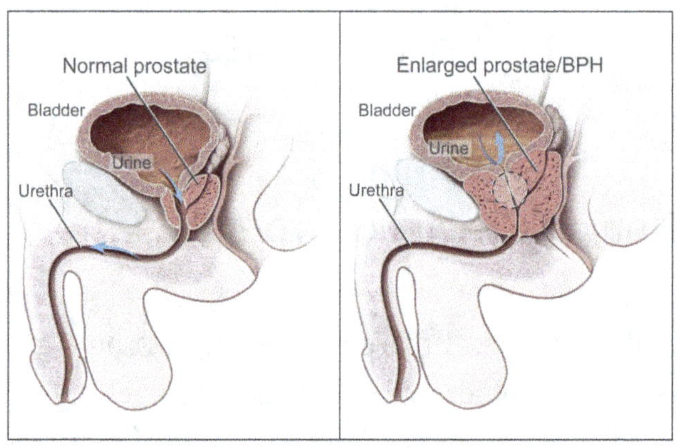

Signs of Trouble

You'll notice changes when your prostate acts up. You might have to really strain to start peeing. Your stream might dribble weakly or even spray. You feel like your bladder doesn't empty all the way. Night trips to the bathroom increase because your bladder gets irritated easily. Leaks can happen too when you laugh or exercise. Pretty soon you dread going anywhere without a bathroom nearby!

What Helps

Don't just live with the nuisance. See your doctor to check what's going on. There are good medication options now that relax muscles near your prostate and bladder neck to improve flow. For some men, minor procedures done in the doctor's office can trim excess prostate tissue pressing on your urethra. Easy solutions exist so ask for help instead of crossing your legs! Try to cut out nighttime liquids, caffeine, and booze too since they send your bladder into overdrive.

Stay positive! BPH is so common now, that there's no reason to suffer through days of difficult peeing. Speak up and take care of this fixable issue.

An enlarged prostate, known medically as benign prostatic hyperplasia (BPH), is very common in aging men. The prostate sits below the bladder and surrounds the urethra, the tube that carries urine. As the prostate grows bigger, it can constrict urine flow and cause problems like:

- Frequent or urgent need to urinate
- Trouble starting a urine stream
- Dribbling after urination ends
- Interrupted sleep to urinate
- Decreased flow strength

BPH is not cancerous but the symptoms can disrupt daily life. There are various enlarged prostate treatment options to consider.

Medications

There are several types of medicines used to shrink prostate tissue and relax muscles around the urethra to improve urine flow.

Alpha-blockers: Help relax bladder neck muscles and muscle fibers in the prostate. This allows urine to flow more easily.

5-alpha reductase inhibitors: Block production of dihydrotestosterone (DHT), a hormone contributing to prostate growth.

Combination drugs: Both alpha-blockers and 5ARIs may be prescribed to maximally improve urine flow and reduce prostate size at the same time.

Interventional Procedures

There are a few common procedures used to treat BPH prostate enlargement by removing excess prostate tissue that's blocking urine flow:

Transurethral needle ablation (TUNA): Radio waves transmitted through needles burn away prostate tissue. Performed with local anesthesia on an outpatient basis.

Transurethral resection of the prostate (TURP): Excess prostate tissue surgically removed to widen the urethra. This is the most common BPH procedure. Typically requires the use of general or spinal anesthesia and 1–2-day hospital stay.

Laser surgery: Laser energy delivery to destroy prostate tissue causing obstruction. Newest technique with the quickest recovery times but precision is essential.

Prostate stents: Tiny metal or plastic tubes implanted in the urethra to keep it open for improved urinary flow.

Minimally invasive treatments like TUNA and laser vaporization lead to fewer bleeding risks and shorter recovery than traditional TURP surgery. Not all treatments work for every man though.

Managing Enlarged Prostate Symptoms

Besides getting medical treatment, some helpful ways to better manage enlarged prostate symptoms in your daily life include:

- Take medications as prescribed and at regular intervals
- Pace your fluid intake, cutting back at least a few hours before bed
- Avoid caffeine and alcohol which can irritate the bladder
- Double void to urinate again if your bladder feels full soon after

- Schedule bathroom trips instead of waiting for urgent feelings
- Try triggers like perineal pressure point tapping to force reluctant urination as needed.

Tracking your symptoms and responses to remedies can help determine what works best for your individual needs. Don't hesitate to discuss persistent issues with your doctor either.

Preventing Aggravation of Symptoms
Some key ways to help prevent aggravating your BPH symptoms include:

- Stay active with regular exercise
- Achieve and maintain a healthy weight
- Follow your doctor's treatment recommendations diligently
- Take medications as prescribed
- Avoid sudden slacking of treatment routine
- Practice stress relaxation techniques
- Attend routine medical checkups for monitoring

Work with your health providers to explore all options and determine which enlarged prostate treatment plan is optimal for managing your symptoms in the long run. Consistent use of medications, healthy lifestyle changes, and medical follow-up are key for the best control.

Chapter 4

Prostate cancer prevention

Lowering Your Risk

Prostate cancer is one of the most common cancers affecting men today. About 1 in 8 men will be diagnosed in their lifetime. The prostate is a walnut-sized gland that sits below the bladder and surrounds the urethra. The prostate's job is to make fluid that nourishes and protects sperm cells.

When cancer starts in this gland, it usually grows very slowly. In fact, there are often no early warning signs or symptoms. That's why getting screened and making healthy lifestyle choices matter for prevention.

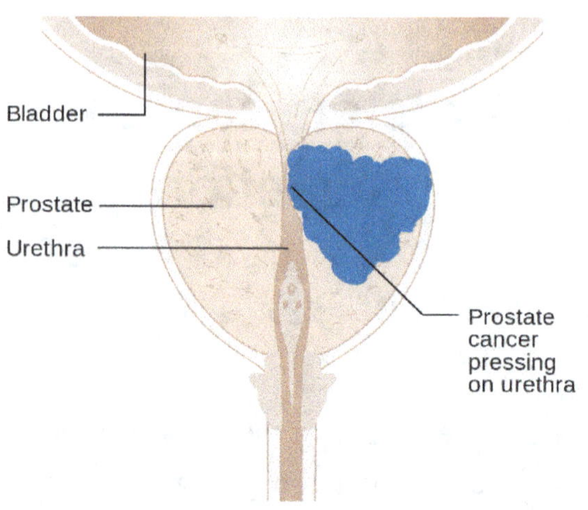

Who's at Risk?

Certain risk factors increase the odds of developing prostate cancer:

- Age: Risk rises dramatically after age 50
- Family history of prostate cancer
- African American ethnicity
- Obesity
- High-fat diet
- Smoking
- Exposure to Agent Orange

However, research also indicates more than 70 percent of prostate cancer cases happen in men with no clear risk factors. That's why preventive measures make good sense for most men.

Prevention Strategies

Ways to lower your personal risk of prostate cancer include:

Get Screened Regularly After Age 50
Most major health organizations recommend men at average risk start getting annual PSA blood tests and physical prostate exams at age 50. Higher-risk men, like those with a family history, should begin screenings at age 45. Early detection gives you the most treatment options with a better outlook. Screening finds over 90% of all prostate cancer cases.

Maintain a Healthy Diet
Eat lots of fruits, vegetables, legumes, whole grains, and healthy fats from nuts, seeds, avocados, and olive oil. Limit processed meat, salty, nitrite-treated foods, and saturated fats.

Making smart, nutritious food choices daily keeps your body and immune defenses functioning at their best.

Stay Active

Shoot for at least 150 minutes per week of vigorous aerobic activity like walking briskly, swimming, biking, or jogging for heart health benefits. Combine this with at least two weekly strength training sessions working major muscle groups. Exercise helps you stay lean and drops your risk of aggressive prostate cancer.

Aim for a Healthy Weight

Carrying excess body fat drives up inflammation, insulin resistance, and sex hormones — all linked to faster prostate cancer development. Steady moderate weight loss combined with routine activity provides protective benefits if you're overweight.

Don't Smoke

Research clearly correlates cigarette smoking with increased prostate cancer mortality rates. Smokers get diagnosed at later stages, are more likely to have a recurrence after treatment, and have lower long-term survival rates. Kicking any tobacco habit is a vital self-care step.

Avoid Harmful Environmental Agents
Minimize exposure to toxic compounds like heavy metals, pesticides, and chemicals used in manufacturing that may have carcinogenic effects. Protective equipment, proper handling, and disposal reduce occupational risk. Water filters provide some home safety against water contaminants.

Address Chronic Inflammation
Managing inflammatory conditions like heart disease and type 2 diabetes also has preventive prostate cancer effects. Anti-inflammatory foods, physical activity, stress relief, and targeted medications all help reduce chronic low-grade inflammation.

Discuss Supplements
Certain vitamins, minerals, and botanicals may help lower prostate cancer risk like vitamin E, selenium, saw palmetto, and green tea extracts. Talk to your doctor before taking any high-dose

supplements for optimal safety and benefits.

Staying proactive with healthy lifestyle
measures and regular screening offers men
increased awareness and better odds of
preventing or catching prostate cancer early.
Keeping your risk lower improves peace of
mind as well as general lifelong health.

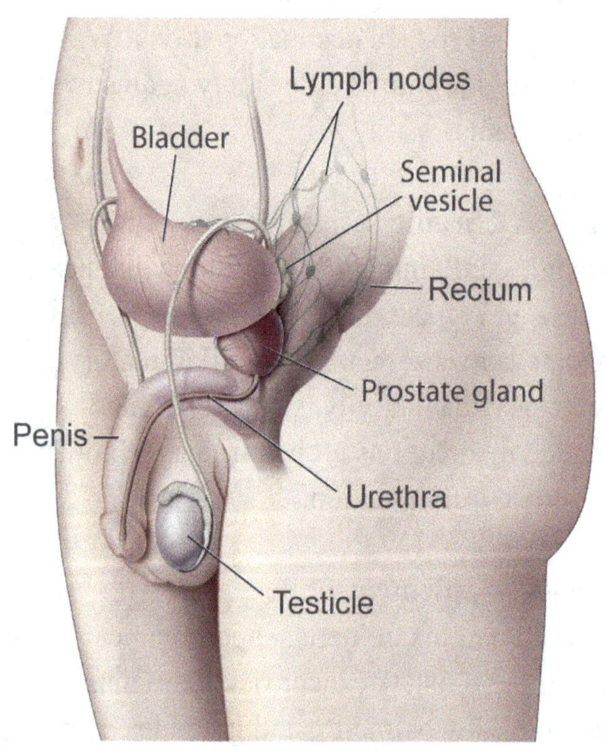

Chapter 5

Prostate health diet

Foods for prostate health

Eating for Optimal Prostate Health

Good nutrition provides key building blocks for overall wellness as well as specific prostate health benefits for men. Making certain healthy foods routine parts of your daily diet can help keep your prostate functioning properly. A prostate-friendly eating plan helps prevent common problems like prostate cancer, enlarged prostate, and prostatitis.

The Prostate Gland and Potential Problems
First understanding what the prostate gland does aids in selecting the best nutrients for this walnut-sized organ. Located under the bladder surrounding the urethra, the prostate produces a thin, milky fluid that:

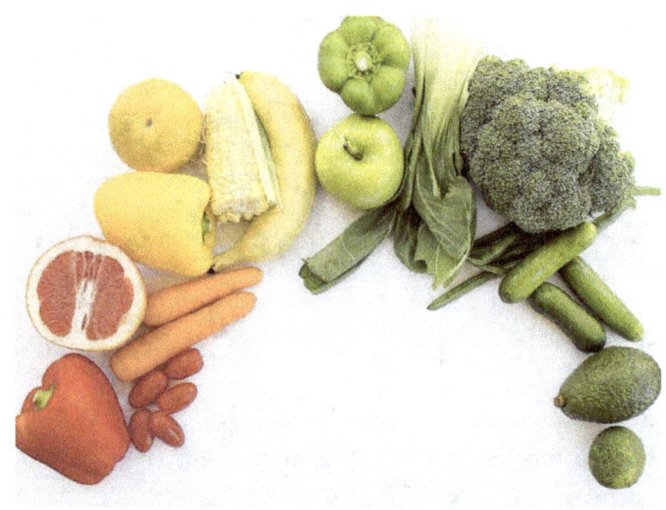

- Protects and nourishes sperm
- Activates sperm movement
- Allows sperm-safe transport in semen

When functioning properly, the prostate fluid assists male fertility capacity. But several issues can arise, especially as a man ages, including:

- Prostate cancer: abnormal cell growth forms tumors impacting health
- Enlarged prostate: benign prostate hyperplasia causes urinary problems

- Prostatitis: prostate tissue swelling leads to genitourinary pain

Fortunately, consuming the right healing and protective foods can aid the prostate.

Top Food Choices for Prostate Health

The best diet plan emphasizes predominantly plant-based anti-inflammatory foods like:

Fruits and Vegetables
Vibrant produce is packed with antioxidants. Lycopene in tomatoes/sauces and cruciferous veggies guard prostate cells. Berries' anthocyanins curb inflammation while citrus vitamin C fortifies immunity to infections causing prostatitis.

Legumes and Soy Foods
Beans and soy, like tofu and edamame, are high in isoflavones. These compounds inhibit testosterone conversion to DHT implicated in enlarged prostates and cancer. Soy also contains genistein, protecting prostate cells from turning malignant.

Nuts and Seeds

Pumpkin, flax, chia, and sesame seeds as well as walnuts, almonds, and peanuts are nutrient powerhouses. Their healthy fats, like omega-3s, bring anti-inflammatory, hormone-balancing benefits. Zinc and selenium minerals in many nuts boost prostate health too.

Green Tea

Packed with protective catechins and epigallocatechin gallate (EGCG), antioxidant-rich green tea guards prostate cells against damage contributing to cancer development. Three or more daily cups are ideal.

Whole Grains

Fiber-rich whole grain breads, oats, brown rice, and quinoa help rid the body of excess hormones and toxins, keeping inflammation in check. Folate in whole grains may also deter prostate cancer progression.

Healthy Fats and Oils Instead of Saturated/Trans Fats

Olive oil, avocado oil, and liquid plant omega oils like flaxseed provide healthy fats that reduce inflammation versus meat, butter, and shortening sources. Using olive and avocado oils on salads and veggies boosts prostate-vital antioxidant absorption too.

Lean Meats (Unless Vegetarian/Vegan)
Rounding out plant-based meals with occasional skinless poultry, fish/shellfish, and grass-fed beef supplies beneficial protein, iron, and zinc too. Choosing lean cuts reduces saturated fats.

Stay Hydrated with Water
Water, black tea, green tea, and low-sugar juices and smoothies keep cells throughout the body and prostate optimally hydrated for nutrient delivery and waste removal functions.

As an extra precaution, limit processed foods, sugars, sweets, and excess alcohol. Aiming for mostly antioxidant-rich plant foods boosts prostate health protection every day through all life stages. Check with your physician about any concerning symptoms and whether specific supplements may provide added benefit too.

Chapter 6

Prostate Massage Benefits

The Benefits of Prostate Massage Therapy

The prostate is a small gland located between the penis and bladder in men. It produces fluid that nourishes and transports sperm. As men age, the prostate tends to grow larger and can cause uncomfortable urinary symptoms. Prostate massage has been used for centuries to promote better prostate health and function.

What is Prostate Massage Therapy?

Prostate massage or prostate milking involves applying gentle pressure to the prostate gland to help drain fluid through the urethra. It may be done internally through the rectum or externally by stimulating the perineum. Prostate massage aims to:

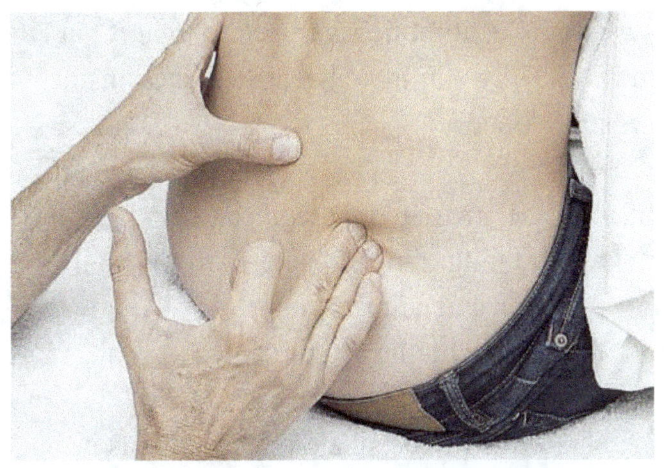

- Relieve prostate congestion
- Reduce inflammation
- Improve prostate secretions
- Support better bladder emptying
- Enhance blood flow

This technique can provide therapeutic benefits for several common prostate issues. Always have it performed by a doctor or trained therapist.

Benefits for Prostatitis

Prostatitis refers to prostate gland swelling and inflammation, often due to a bacterial infection.

This causes painful urinary and ejaculation symptoms. Antibiotics are used to treat it but may not fully eliminate bacteria tucked inside prostate tissues.

In this case, prostate massage can help by:
- Draining trapped bacteria from small ducts and acini
- Improving the effectiveness of oral antibiotics if combined
- Reducing the size of calcifications or prostate stones
- Slowing formations of prostate cysts.

The increase in genitourinary blood circulation can also help resolve inflammation.

Benefits for Enlarged Prostate

Many men develop benign prostatic hyperplasia (BPH) as they age, causing prostate enlargement pressing on the urethra. This leads to increased urinary frequency, urgency, and stopping or starting urine stream issues.

Gentle and thorough periodic prostate massage provides BPH symptom relief through:

- Removing pooled prostatic secretions to unblock urethra
- Improving muscle tone in sphincters and pelvic floor
- Strengthening bladder control
- Reducing residual urine volumes
- It also slows prostate overgrowth and may help avoid eventual surgery.

Benefits for Erectile Dysfunction

Achieving erections requires proper blood flow and muscular coordination. As the small arteries surrounding the prostate grow constricted, it reduces vital blood movement to and from erectile tissues. Limited circulation causes chronic fluid buildup too.

Prostate massage aids erectile strength by:

- Widening compressed vessels to boost vascular flow
- Increasing blood movement to the genital region
- Reducing internal prostate congestion

- Strengthening pelvic muscles involved in erections
- This boosts nutrition delivery for stronger rigidity.

For the greatest safety and therapeutic effectiveness, prostate massage therapy is best performed by a doctor or qualified specialist using proper simple medical equipment in a clinical setting. Results improve significantly with multiple recurring treatment sessions.

Combined with other therapies like diet changes, stress reduction, medications, or herbal supplements, regular prostate massage offers multiple benefits supporting better prostate drainage and urinary tract functionality.

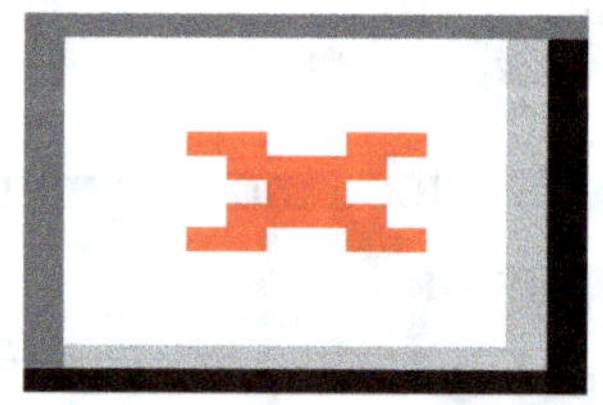

Chapter 7

Prostate Cancer Surgery

Understanding Prostate Cancer Surgery Options

When prostate cancer is detected early while still confined to the prostate gland, surgery to remove the cancerous tissue may be an effective treatment option. There are several types of prostate cancer surgery with the intent of eradicating detectable cancer in the prostate.

Reasons for Choosing Surgery

Surgery allows thorough removal of localized cancer cells within the prostate before they can spread to other areas. Reasons you may opt for prostate cancer surgery when eligible include:

- High cure rates for early-stage prostate cancer via surgery
- Eliminates the need for frequent PSA screening afterward

- May reduce the risk of side effects that accompany radiation
- Often recommended for younger patients for better quality of life

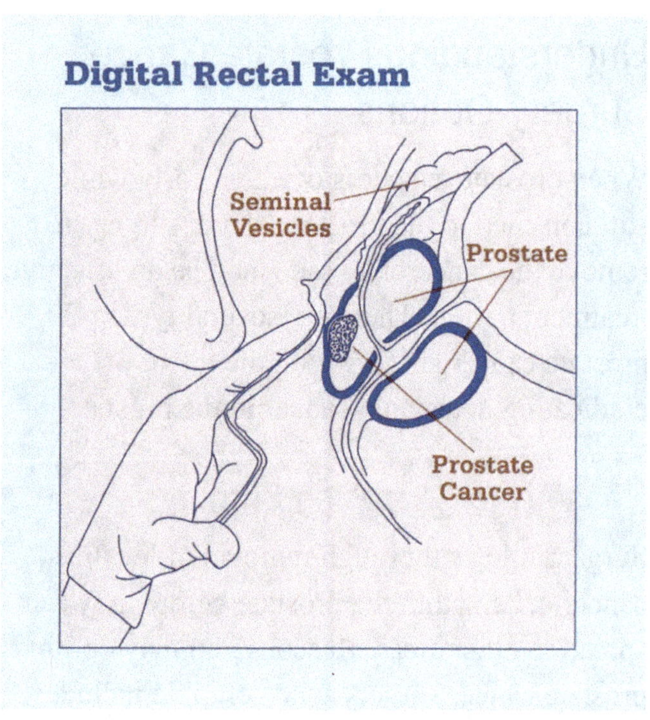

Research shows favorable long-term survival rates.

Of course, personal considerations regarding recovery time, potential surgical complications, and side effects like incontinence or erectile dysfunction influence the treatment decision as well. Your doctor will discuss the pros and cons with you.

Popular Prostate Surgery Approaches

Common types of prostate cancer surgery include:

Radical Prostatectomy
This common procedure removes the entire prostate gland plus surrounding tissue. It's done as open surgery through a sizable lower abdomen incision, or via minimally invasive laparoscopic or robotic keyhole surgery requiring smaller cuts. Each way is highly effective at eliminating cancer if it hasn't spread beyond the prostate.

Nerve-Sparing Prostatectomy
Using microscopic magnification, surgeons carefully dissect free and preserve delicate nerves involved in erectile function surrounding the prostate instead of cutting them. This nerve-sparing technique greatly reduces the risk of post-surgical impotence, especially for

appropriate younger patients with early, very
low-risk cancer diagnoses. Not all cases allow
nerves to be spared though.

Cryosurgery or Cryoablation
Guided imaging lets surgeons insert small
probes into the precise prostate tumor area
detected via prior biopsy. Liquid nitrogen
applied through the probes forms ice balls that
freeze and kill cancerous tissues while
protecting other interior prostate gland tissues
and structures. No incisions means faster
recovery but later prostate tissue death and
shedding can cause temporary side effects.

High-Intensity Focused Ultrasound (HIFU)
The latest non-invasive surgical option uses
tightly focused ultrasound waves directed only
at identified cancer lesions within the prostate
based on MRI images during the procedure. The
intense heat destroys tumors but doesn't impact
tissues in the pathway to the target area. Done
as an outpatient procedure, favorable short-term
results for low-risk prostate tumors make this a
promising newer approach.

Talk to your urologic oncology team about which prostate cancer surgery technique may be optimal for your situation. Gather all the facts so you comprehend limitations, side effect risks, and projected outcomes. For men undergoing surgical removal of early prostate cancer, the future prognosis is generally quite positive.

Prostate Cancer Survival Rates by Stage:

Prostate Cancer Staging and Survival Rates Prostate cancer is one of the most common cancers among men. **According to the American Cancer Society, about 1 in 8 men will be diagnosed with prostate cancer at some point during their lifetime.** Staging prostate cancer is important to determine the best treatment options and to assess the chances of survival.

What is Staging?

Staging describes the extent of the cancer in the body. It is based on the size and spread of the tumor, whether cancer has spread to lymph nodes or other organs, and certain other factors.

Determining the stage of prostate cancer relies on results from diagnostic tests like biopsies, imaging scans, and blood tests. Knowing the stage also helps doctors estimate survival statistics and determine the most appropriate treatments.

The 5-Year Survival Rates by Stage
Stage 1 - The cancer is small and localized only to the prostate gland. It has not spread to lymph nodes or elsewhere in the body. The 5-year relative survival rate for stage 1 prostate cancer is close to 100%.

Stage 2 - The tumor may be larger and there may be some abnormal cells around the prostate, but the cancer is still confined to the prostate. Stage 2 prostate cancer has a 5-year relative survival rate of nearly 100%.

Stage 3 - The cancer has grown outside the prostate gland and may have spread to the seminal vesicles, but not yet reached the lymph nodes, bones, or other organs. The 5-year survival rate drops slightly to about 93%.

Stage 4 - This means the prostate cancer has spread beyond the seminal vesicles to nearby tissues like the bladder, colon, lymph nodes, bones, liver, or lungs. Stage 4 has a 5-year relative survival rate of around 30%.

Within some stages, some subcategories provide more details about how far the cancer has spread. For example, Stage 3A vs 3B, or Stage 4A vs 4B. The further along in the substages, generally the lower the survival rates within that primary stage category.

Factors Affecting Survival Rates

The stage of prostate cancer at diagnosis has the biggest impact on a man's outlook, but several other factors also affect individual survival rates, including:

- The man's age at diagnosis
- His Gleason score based on biopsy results
- His PSA levels

- Any gene mutations or tumor markers identified
- His response to initial prostate cancer treatment
- His general health apart from the cancer

Younger men with early-stage low to intermediate-risk prostate cancer have better odds for long-term survival. Older men diagnosed at later stages may have lower chances for a cure.

Importance of Early Detection

Early prostate cancer often causes no signs or symptoms which is why screening is essential to detect it when it's most treatable. Men at average risk should have discussions with their doctor beginning at age 45-50 about prostate cancer testing so it can be diagnosed at an early stage if present. Catching it early while still localized gives men the widest range of treatment options and the greatest odds of survival.

The future for men with prostate cancer continues to improve with advances in surgical techniques, radiation therapies, chemotherapy drugs, and more. Researchers are hard at work trying to develop better diagnostic methods and more effective treatments to increase survival and improve the quality of life for prostate cancer patients.

Chapter 8

Prostate Cancer Research Advances

The Latest in Prostate Cancer Research

Prostate cancer is one of the most common cancers occurring in men. Thankfully mortality rates are declining as research reveals more effective diagnostic and treatment options. Scientists work continuously to improve early detection and develop innovative new therapies for better survival outcomes.

Advancing PSA Testing

The PSA (prostate-specific antigen) blood test remains the standard screening method to indicate prostate issues. However, PSA levels can be elevated due to noncancerous prostate enlargement also.

Ongoing research to enhance PSA testing

accuracy includes evaluating PSA fluctuations over time, PSA density adjustments, and combining it with other protein biomarkers found through patient genome mapping and sophisticated risk calculators. More accurate analysis aims to reduce unnecessary prostate biopsies.

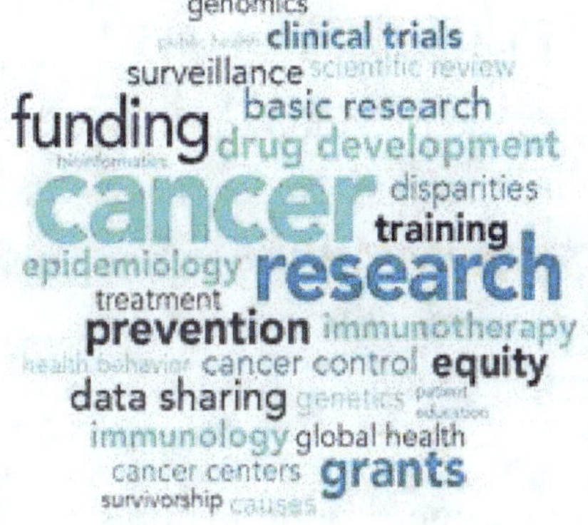

Enhancing Biopsy Accuracy

Collecting several tissue samples through transrectal ultrasound-guided biopsies is the standard way abnormal PSA levels get investigated further. However, this method can still miss some cancers.

To improve accuracy, researchers are studying advanced color Doppler imaging to visualize prostate lesions better during sampling. Fusing MRI and ultrasound offers enhanced guidance too. New biomarkers identified in urine or blood could provide less invasive early diagnostic abilities as well.

Refining Risk Stratification

Multiple genetic mutation tracking tools allow more precise prostate cancer risk assessment now. These include genes like BRCA1/BRCA2, HOXB13, and variations in RNA microstructures within tumors.

Identifying unique genetic features of each man's cancer helps predict accurate aggression risk levels and responses for optimizing treatment personalization. This is called precision oncology.

Evaluating Active Surveillance Advancements

Active surveillance simply means closely tracking early, low-risk prostate cancer growth parameters over time rather than rushing aggressive treatments. This spares treatment side effects unless warranted later by quicker changes.

Adding advanced imaging and biomarkers to standard PSA monitoring is being studied to improve active surveillance safety and criteria guidance. Enhanced MRI now detects tumors missed on biopsies too. Allowing men to delay interventions remains a priority.

Exploring Newer Treatment Innovations
Beyond surgery, radiation and chemotherapy advancements aim to reduce side effects and extend survival. Some key areas include:

- High-intensity focused ultrasound to ablate tumors

- Cryosurgery freezing for low-risk cancers
- Nanotechnology to deliver targeted cell toxins
- Cancer vaccines and drugs to spark anti-tumor immunity
- Robotic surgery refinements
- Proton beam therapy to destroy growths without harming surrounding tissue
- Combination therapies for high-risk prostate cancer
- Immunotherapy drugs to unleash the body's own defenses

The future looks bright when it comes to expanding early detection and treatment choices for prostate cancer patients through dedicated ongoing research.

Radiation Therapy Prostate Cancer

Understanding Radiation Treatment for Prostate Cancer

Radiation therapy is an effective treatment for prostate cancer especially in the early stages when it is still confined to the prostate gland. Radiation aims a beam of intense energy at tumor cells destroying their ability to grow and multiply. It offers a viable alternative or addition to surgery to reach and eliminate cancer.

Goals of Radiation Therapy

The major goals of radiation for prostate cancer are to:

- Shrink the size of a tumor before surgery
- Slow down or halt tumor growth when surgery is not indicated
- Kill cancer cells lingering post-surgery to reduce risk of recurrence
- Eradicate all cancer cells entirely for some mid and low-risk tumors
- Provide relief from advanced prostate cancer symptoms when the disease has progressed
- Reduce pain and other issues from metastasized cancer spread to the bones

Types of Radiation Therapy Used

There are two main categories of radiation therapy:

External Beam Radiation
-Use of a machine to beam focused radiation waves at the tumor from outside the body. Common external techniques include 3D conformal radiation, intensity-modulated radiation (IMRT), and proton beam therapy. Most men get external radiation at cancer centers five days a week for several weeks.

Internal Radiation (Brachytherapy)
-Includes inserting radioactive implant seeds or ribbons directly into the prostate gland tissue. Low-dose radioactive iodine, palladium or cesium seed implants deliver targeted radiation over months, with no further treatment needed.

Potential Side Effects

Radiation therapy typically lasts anywhere from 1 to 9 weeks. Acute side effects during the weeks of treatment can involve rectal issues like bowel irritation, bladder problems with painful/frequent urination, and for short periods erectile dysfunction.

Some long-term side effects of radiation may include:

- Chronic proctitis - rectal inflammation, pain, bleeding
- Cystitis - inflammation of the bladder lining causing painful urination
- Loss of fertility due to sperm damage
- Loss of erectile function long-term

Close follow-up care includes symptom management strategies and physical therapy for any late-onset effects after finishing radiation.

Advantages of Radiation Therapy for Prostate Cancer:

- Effective non-invasive treatment for early cancers
- Eradicates cancer without incisions or hospital stays for external radiation

- Allows men to maintain a good quality of life during and after therapy
- Lower risk of incontinence struggles than surgery
- Brachytherapy limits radiation exposure to healthy tissues

Discuss all prostate cancer treatment options thoroughly with your physicians so you can determine if radiation or a combination of radiation and surgical methods is optimal. With so many types of radiation therapy available, most men receive highly successful results.

Chapter 9

Living with Prostate Cancer: Coping Strategies and Support

Being diagnosed with prostate cancer can be very scary and overwhelming. You may be feeling many different emotions like fear, anger, sadness, or anxiety about what lies ahead. These feelings are completely normal.

Prostate cancer is one of the most common types of cancer in men. When caught early, it is often very treatable. However, dealing with prostate cancer and its treatment can still be highly stressful for both patients and their loved ones.

Coping with the Physical Effects

Prostate cancer itself often causes no symptoms at first. However, treatments like surgery, radiation, hormone therapy, and chemotherapy can lead to difficult physical side effects. These may include incontinence, erectile dysfunction, fatigue, nausea, and bowel issues among others.

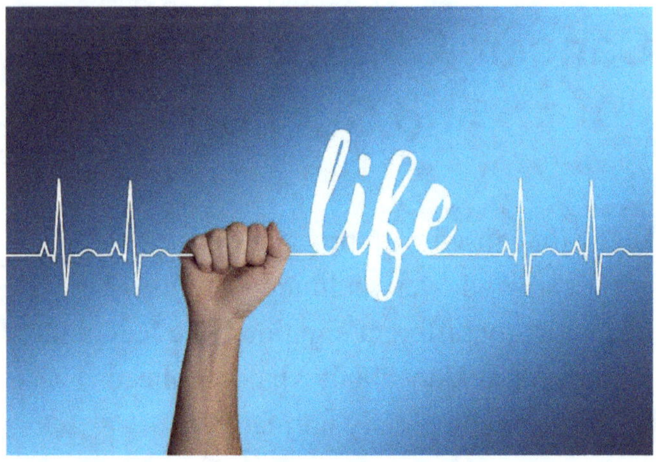

It's important to communicate openly with your doctor about any side affects you experience. There are often medications or techniques that can help manage these issues. You should also take good care of yourself through proper nutrition, exercise as you are able, and getting enough rest.

Handling the Emotional Impact

In addition to the physical effects, prostate cancer can take a big emotional toll. Many men say they experience depression, anxiety, fear of the unknown, and struggles with their self-image and sense of masculinity.

Don't try to face these alone. Seek support from loved ones who can listen and provide comfort and encouragement. You may also benefit from joining a prostate cancer support group. Speaking to a counselor or therapist can also help process the complex emotions around cancer.

Getting the Right Support

When going through prostate cancer, having the proper support system in place is vital. This may include:

- Loved ones like a spouse, family, and close friends who can help with practicalities, be a sounding board, and provide companionship
- A doctor and medical team you trust and can communicate openly with about all aspects of your care

- Prostate cancer support communities, whether online or local in-person groups
- Counseling or therapy to help process emotions around your diagnosis
- Workplace understanding about needing time off for treatments and medical appointments
- Help with things like transportation, meals, chores, and childcare as needed during treatments

Though the prostate cancer journey is challenging, it's important to be proactive in getting the physical and emotional support you need. Don't be afraid to ask for help. With resilience and the right care, many men can thrive during and after prostate cancer.

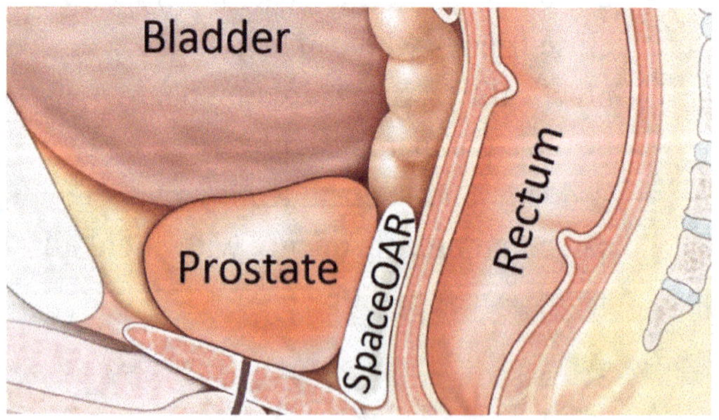

Chapter 10

Integrative Approaches: Nutrition, Exercise, and Mind-Body Connection

When dealing with a major health issue like cancer, taking an integrative approach can be very beneficial. This means looking at your whole person - mind, body, and spirit - and finding many different ways to nurture healing.

Traditional medical treatments are incredibly important. However, adding in healthy lifestyle practices and mind-body techniques can also play a big supportive role. Let's explore some key integrative strategies:

Nutrition for Healing

What you eat can be powerful medicine. A balanced, nutrient-rich diet full of fruits, vegetables, lean proteins, and healthy fats gives your body the fuel it needs to stay strong during treatment.

Some foods are especially good for fighting cancer and managing treatment side effects. These include foods high in antioxidants like berries, tomatoes, leafy greens, fatty fish, nuts, and seeds. Probiotic foods like yogurt, garlic, onions, and fermented items can also be helpful.

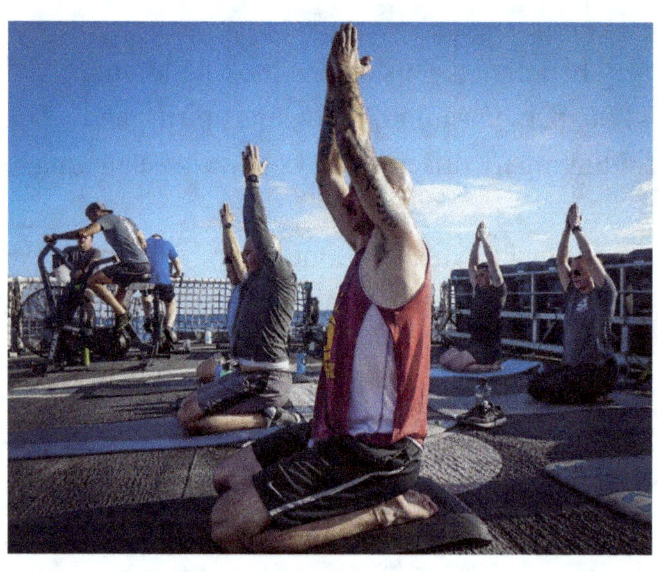

Exercise for Strength

Being physically active can improve energy

levels, build strength and endurance, lift your mood, and reduce stress. Gentle exercise like walking, yoga, or swimming may be beneficial, depending on your treatment plan.

Even light movement throughout the day, such as marching in place or doing basic strength exercises from a chair or bed, can make a big difference. Be sure to follow your doctor's exercise recommendations and listen to your body.

Mind-Body for Resilience

Managing thoughts, beliefs, emotions, and stress levels is a huge part of holistic care. Practices like meditation, guided imagery, art therapy, journaling, and breathing exercises can provide powerful mind-body benefits.

Things like support groups, counseling or therapy, spiritual practices, and spending time in nature can also nurture resilience. Do what resonates best to calm your mind, process emotions, and stay hopeful and motivated.

Integrative Promotes Thriving

An integrative care approach helps nurture your total well-being during health challenges. Making good nutrition, physical activity, and mind-body practices part of your healing strategy can maximize your quality of life.

Be sure to partner with your medical providers and let them guide you in making wise integrative choices that provide safe, effective support. With innovative treatments combined with healthy integrative elements, you can thrive through cancer and beyond.

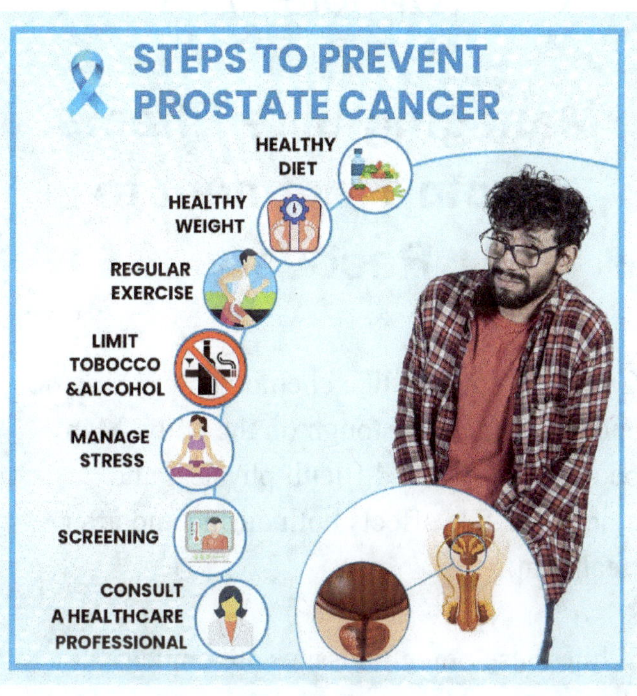

STEPS TO PREVENT PROSTATE CANCER
HEALTHY DIET
HEALTHY WEIGHT
REGULAR EXERCISE
LIMIT TOBOCCO &ALCOHOL
MANAGE STRESS
SCREENING
CONSULT A HEALTHCARE PROFESSIONAL

Chapter 11

Managing Side Effects: From Treatment to Recovery

Cancer treatments like chemotherapy, radiation, and surgery can be tough on the body. Many people experience difficult physical and emotional side effects both during and after treatment.

While these potential issues are unpleasant, there are ways to prevent and manage side effects so you can stay as comfortable as possible on your healing journey.

Common Side Effects

Different treatments lead to various side effects. Some of the most frequent include:

- Fatigue and sleep issues
- Nausea and vomiting

- Appetite loss and weight changes
- Hair loss
- Mouth sores
- Skin rashes or burns
- Nerve pain and numbness
- Lymphedema (fluid buildup)
- Fertility issues
- Anxiety, depression, and "chemo brain" (cognitive changes)

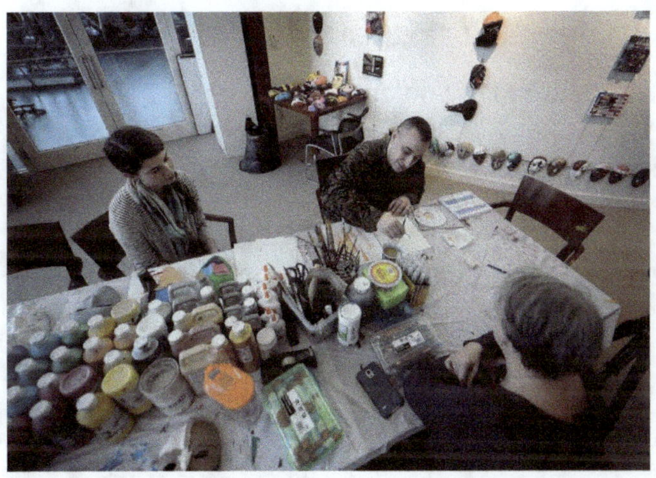

Open Communication Helps

One of the best ways to handle side effects is through clear communication with your medical team. Be upfront in describing any new symptoms or problems you experience. Don't try to tough it out, as your doctors can provide medications, remedies, and coping techniques.

Track your side effects carefully and discuss management strategies at every appointment. Also ask what short-term and long-term effects could arise so you know what to watch for.

Strategies for Relief

There are many potential remedies for side effect relief, such as:

- Anti-nausea and pain medications
- Nutritional drinks and supplements
- Gentle exercises and physical therapy
- Acupuncture and massage
- Support groups and counseling
- Occupational therapy for regaining abilities

Your doctor may recommend an integrative approach using combinations of medications, therapies, and lifestyle strategies. Be open to different techniques to find what provides you the most relief and comfort.

The Recovery Process

For most, side effects gradually ease after cancer treatments end. However, some may have longer-lasting issues requiring continued management and rehabilitation.

It's important to be patient during the recovery process and celebrate small daily wins. Lean on your support network, and keep prioritizing practices like adequate rest, good nutrition, hydration, and gentle exercise as you're able.

With time, self-care and the right strategies in place, the goal is to regain your full strength and vitality. If you face persistent problems, seek further medical help. Managing side effects is key to feeling your best through every stage of healing.

Chapter 12

The Role of Mental Health in Prostate Cancer Survival

When dealing with prostate cancer, focusing on physical health is crucial. However, mental, and emotional well-being also plays a major role in recovery and survival.

A prostate cancer diagnosis can lead to many difficult emotions like fear, anger, sadness, and anxiety. How well a person copes with these feelings can greatly impact their overall quality of life and treatment outcomes.

The Mind-Body Connection

There is a strong link between our minds and bodies when it comes to health. High levels of psychological distress have been shown to weaken the immune system's ability to fight disease. Stress also influences inflammation levels, which can affect cancer progression.

On the other hand, maintaining a positive mindset strengthens resilience and healing ability. A prostate cancer patient who practices stress management, counseling, support groups, or other therapies tends to have lower rates of anxiety and depression.

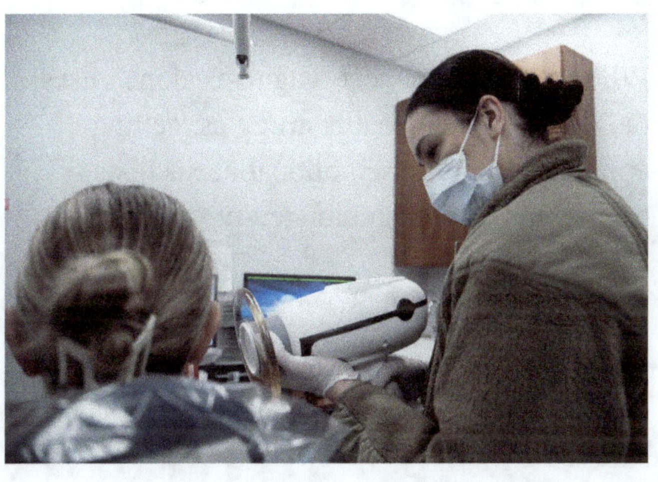

Better Mental Health, Better Survival

Multiple research studies have found that prostate cancer patients with good mental health and lower distress levels have higher survival rates compared to those with more anxiety and depression.

One key study followed over 40,000 pairs of prostate cancer patients and found that the men with available mental health support and fewer untreated mental health issues lived significantly longer. In fact, their survival rates increased by nearly 30% over 18 years.

While a prostate cancer diagnosis alone raises the risk of mental health struggles, getting appropriate care for emotional needs boosts overall well-being and longevity.

Finding the Right Support

There are many ways to nurture mental and emotional strength when facing prostate cancer, such as:

- Individual counseling or therapy to process difficult thoughts and feelings
- Couples or family counseling to improve communication and closeness

- Support groups with others going through similar experiences
- Stress management techniques like meditation, yoga, deep breathing
- Enjoyable hobbies and activities that promote a sense of normalcy
- Maintaining social connections and avoiding isolation

Mental health support looks different for everyone. The key is finding healthy coping strategies that provide comfort and meaning. With resilience on both the physical and psychological side, many men can thrive on their prostate cancer journey.

Chapter 13

Beyond the Diagnosis: Life After Prostate Cancer

Getting a prostate cancer diagnosis can be one of the scariest experiences of a man's life. However, with improved treatment options, the future is becoming brighter for many patients.

After going through therapy, surgery, or other treatments, the reality of life after cancer may start to set in. While this "new normal" brings its own challenges, it also opens the door to a renewed outlook and deeper appreciation for health.

Managing Lasting Effects

Depending on the stage and treatments used, some men face longer-term side effects and adjustments, such as:

- Fatigue and insomnia

- Urinary or bowel incontinence
- Loss of sexual function/erectile dysfunction
- Hormonal changes and weight gain
- Lymphedema (fluid buildup) and neuropathy (nerve pain)
- Anxiety, depression, "chemo brain" (cognitive issues)

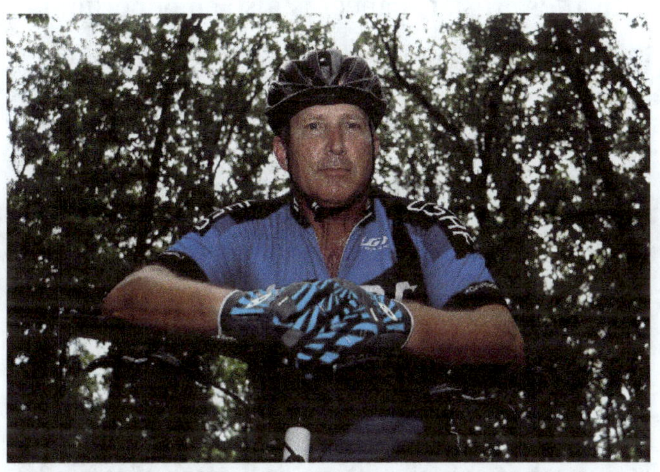

While frustrating, many of these lingering effects can be managed through medications, lifestyle changes, counseling, rehab programs, or additional treatments. Having open conversations with your doctor about any lasting problems is important.

Embracing Lifestyle Changes

In the wake of cancer, making positive health behavior changes becomes even more crucial. A balanced diet full of cancer-fighting nutrients, regular physical activity, stress management, and weight control may reduce the risk of recurrence.

Life after prostate cancer is also an opportunity to reevaluate priorities. Some men may decide to spend more quality time with loved ones, take up enjoyable hobbies, deepen their spirituality, or make other meaningful life adjustments.

Finding Purpose and Support

A cancer experience can feel like loss – of health, of confidence, of former identities. However, it can also serve as a catalyst to find new purpose, passions, and self-knowledge.

Joining a support group allows connecting with others who understand what you've gone through. Many men also find empowerment in becoming prostate cancer advocates, funders of research, or peer supporters to newly diagnosed patients.

73

Moving Forward with Resilience

Although no one wishes for a cancer diagnosis, the journey can shape perspectives in powerful ways. With resilience and the right care team, men can regain their quality of life and appreciate every day in a profound new light.

If you're struggling, don't be afraid to ask for help from loved ones, doctors, mental health professionals, or local cancer support resources. With comprehensive care addressing body, mind, and spirit, it is very possible to thrive beyond prostate cancer.

Chapter 14

Prevention Strategies: Promoting Prostate Health for a Lifetime

Prostate cancer is one of the most common cancers in men. While some risk factors like age, genetics, and race are out of our control, there are many positive lifestyle steps guys can take to reduce their risk and stay prostate healthy.

The prostate is a small gland located below the bladder in men. Its main function is producing fluid that nourishes and transports sperm. Keeping the prostate in good shape through prevention strategies is ideal.

Diet and Nutrition

What you eat plays a major role in prostate health. A nutritious diet filled with fruits, vegetables, whole grains, lean proteins, and

healthy fats promotes overall vitality.
Some foods provide extra prostate benefits:

- Tomatoes and pink grapefruit contain the antioxidant lycopene
- Green tea and turmeric have anti-inflammatory properties
- Fatty fishlike salmon and sardines provide omega-3s
- Cruciferous veggies like broccoli may help regulate testosterone levels

Staying hydrated by drinking enough water daily is also ideal.

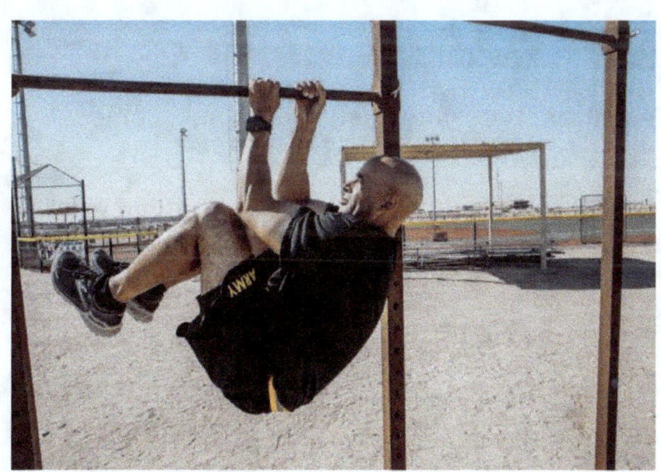

Active Lifestyle

Regular exercise is another key prevention factor. Obesity raises prostate cancer risk, so maintaining a healthy weight through diet and physical activity is wise.

Aim for at least 30 minutes of moderate activity most days, such as brisk walking, swimming, or sports. Strength training to build muscle mass can also be protective.

Even small increases in activity levels, like taking movement breaks and avoiding excessive sitting, provide benefits for prostate wellness.

Other Prevention Boosters

Additional prostate health strategies include:

- Not smoking (smokers have higher risk)
- Reducing stress through meditation, yoga, etc.
- Scheduling regular prostate exams/screenings
- Talking to your doctor about medications that may impact prostate health

The Right Preventions Equal Powerful Protection

By combining a nutrient-rich diet, regular exercise, screening tests, and other wholesome lifestyle practices, men can take active steps to significantly lower their chance of developing prostate cancer or other prostate issues down the road.

It's never too early or too late to make prevention a priority. Simple daily choices add up and optimize lifelong vitality and prostate health.

Chapter 15

Advocacy and Awareness: Making a Difference

Being diagnosed with prostate cancer can feel overwhelming. However, many men decide to turn their difficult experience into motivation to make a positive difference. By raising awareness and advocating for better care and resources, these everyday heroes are creating hope and change.

Some get involved with cancer support organizations by volunteering, fundraising, or serving as peer mentors to newly diagnosed patients. Others participate in awareness campaigns and public outreach events to educate communities.

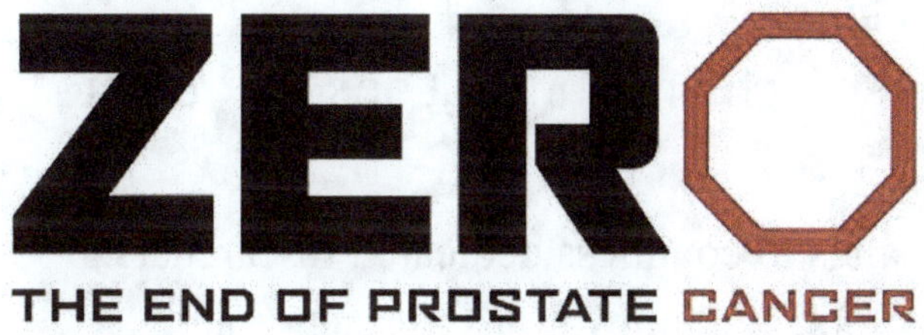

Many survivors use their voices to influence policies and laws around prostate cancer screening, treatment access, and quality of care. They may share their personal journeys with the media, speak at events, or contact government officials.

Even simple actions like wearing advocacy merchandise or using social media to spread facts can have a huge ripple effect. No effort for the cause is too small. Together, prostate cancer advocates create a loud, united voice demanding progress.

Real people putting their passion into action is what drives positive change. Courageous advocates bring vital issues to the forefront and improve many lives.

Research and Innovations in Prostate Cancer

Thanks to countless dedicated researchers, doctors, and innovations in science and technology, the prostate cancer field is rapidly evolving. Many exciting new frontiers are being explored to detect cancer earlier, treat it more precisely and effectively, and enhance patient outcomes and quality of life.

Some key areas of progress include:

- More accurate screening and genetic testing
- Advanced imaging to better visualize tumors
- Targeted radiation therapies that spare healthy tissue
- Immunotherapy treatments that harness the body's own defenses

- Robotic prostate surgery for less invasive procedures
- New medications and hormone therapies with fewer side effects

Researchers are also exploring the potential of lifestyle factors, nutrition, exercise, and complementary therapies in prevention and treatment. With knowledge expanding, more personalized and integrative care plans are possible.

While much work remains, each new discovery builds hope. Progress takes persistence, funding, clinical trials, and courageous patient participants. Thanks to these efforts, the future looks brighter than ever before.

Inspirational Stories: Survivors' Journeys

At the heart of the prostate cancer experience are the survivors themselves - the brave individuals who faced this challenge with resilience, determination, and often unexpected strength.

From their unique personal journeys emerges a mosaic of inspirational stories filled with profound lessons about living every moment fully, cherishing loved ones, and never giving up hope.

One man describes how his diagnosis at an early age shattered his feelings of invincibility yet ultimately revealed his life's purpose in motivating other young survivors. Another shares how the experience became a wake-up call to reprioritize work-life balance and reconnect with passions outside his career.

Many survivors say they gained deeper self-knowledge, appreciation for life's fragility, and the inner fortitude they never knew they possessed until faced with mortality. Surrounded by the unwavering support of their families, friends and care teams, ordinary people achieved extraordinary resilience.

While every prostate cancer journey is different, these inspirational stories collectively symbolize the tenacity of the human spirit. In

their own ways, each survivor's path highlights
the courage to embrace life fully when
confronted by life's greatest challenges.

Chapter 16

The Prostate Health Diet

What to Eat to Prevent and Heal Prostate Problems Including Prostate Cancer, BPH Enlarged Prostate, and Prostatitis

Prostate health is a crucial aspect of overall well-being that often gets overlooked. The significance of maintaining a healthy prostate and explores the role of a well-balanced diet in preventing and healing various prostate problems, including prostate cancer, BPH (enlarged prostate), and prostatitis.

Understanding Prostate Problems

Prostate Cancer

Prostate cancer is a prevalent concern among men, making it imperative to adopt preventive measures. A wholesome diet can significantly contribute to reducing the risk of prostate cancer.

BPH Enlarged Prostate

Benign Prostatic Hyperplasia (BPH) is a common condition affecting aging men. Discover how dietary choices can impact the progression of an enlarged prostate.

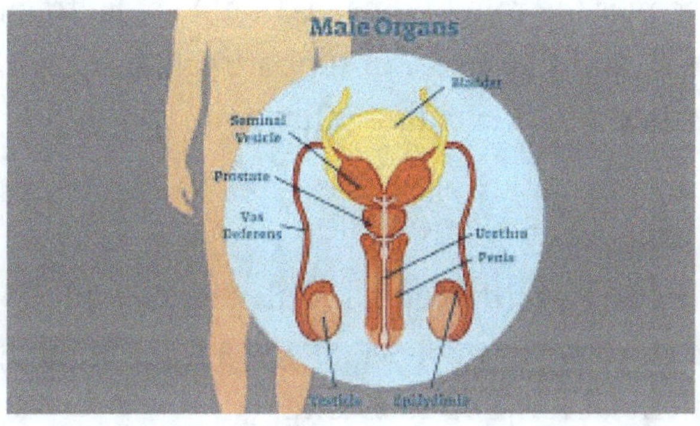

Prostatitis

Inflammation of the prostate, known as prostatitis, can lead to discomfort and pain. Learn about dietary strategies to alleviate symptoms and promote healing.

The Prostate Health Diet

Antioxidant-Rich Foods
Incorporating fruits and vegetables rich in antioxidants can provide protection against cellular damage, benefiting overall prostate health.

Omega-3 Fatty Acids

Discover the role of omega-3 fatty acids, found in fish and flaxseeds, in supporting a healthy prostate and preventing inflammation.

Cruciferous Vegetables

Broccoli, cauliflower, and kale are examples of cruciferous vegetables that contain compounds beneficial for prostate health.

Zinc-Rich Foods

Zinc is a mineral essential for prostate function. Explore foods that are excellent sources of zinc to maintain a well-functioning prostate.

Foods to Avoid

Red and Processed Meats

Excessive consumption of red and processed meats has been linked to an increased risk of prostate issues. Learn about alternative protein sources.

High-Calcium Foods

Balancing calcium intake is crucial, as excessive amounts may contribute to prostate problems. Discover how to manage calcium levels effectively.

Excessive Dairy Consumption

Explore the relationship between dairy consumption and prostate health, with insights into moderation and suitable alternatives.

Hydration and Prostate Health

Importance of Water

Proper hydration plays a role in overall health, including prostate health. Learn about the benefits of adequate water intake.

Limiting Caffeine and Alcohol

Excessive caffeine and alcohol consumption can negatively impact prostate health. Discover moderation strategies for a healthier lifestyle. Lifestyle Changes for Prostate Health

Regular Exercise

Physical activity is not only beneficial for cardiovascular health but also plays a role in supporting a healthy prostate. Explore suitable exercise routines.

Stress Management

Chronic stress can contribute to prostate problems. Learn effective stress management techniques for a balanced and healthy life.

Sleep Hygiene

Quality sleep is crucial for overall well-being. Explore the connection between proper sleep and prostate health.

Recipes for a Prostate-Friendly Diet

Prostate-Boosting Smoothie
Try a delicious smoothie recipe packed with ingredients known for their prostate health benefits.

Salmon and Vegetable Stir-Fry
Discover a tasty and nutritious stir-fry recipe featuring salmon and prostate-friendly vegetables.

Supplements for Prostate Health
Saw Palmetto
Understand the potential benefits of saw palmetto, an herbal supplement often used for prostate health.

Vitamin D
Explore the role of vitamin D in supporting prostate health and methods to ensure adequate intake.

Seeking Professional Advice
Consultation with a Nutritionist
Considering individual health needs, consulting

with a nutritionist can provide personalized
dietary recommendations.

Regular Health Checkups
Regular checkups are essential for detecting and
addressing potential prostate issues early. Learn
about the importance of routine health
assessments.

Success Stories and Testimonials
Real-Life Experiences
Read about individuals who have successfully
improved their prostate health through dietary
changes and lifestyle adjustments.

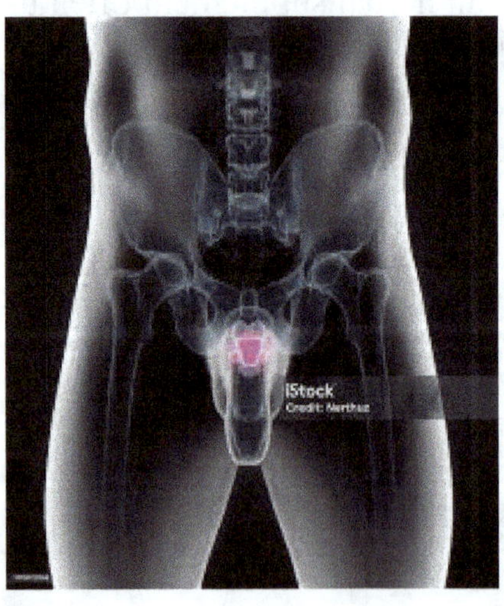

Additionally, adopting a prostate health diet is a proactive approach to preventing and healing various prostate problems. By making informed dietary choices, incorporating exercise, and managing stress, men can enhance their overall well-being and reduce the risk of prostate issues.

Please support with
your valuable positive reviews!
it is highly appreciated.

Please support my other contents here:

DIY Medicinal Gardening.... Click Here!

Thank you